Copyright ©2020 ARNOLD KUNTZ PH.D

CONTENTS

INTRODUCTION

When following a ketogenic diet, it is not uncommon for people to neglect eating quality sources of fiber in an effort to avoid any carbohydrate intake. There is a chance this can lead to constipation, poor digestion, and a lack of certain vitamins and minerals.

In the keto world, there is always controversy among experts when it comes to dirty vs. clean keto, the optimal sources of fat, the optimal carbohydrates, supplements and yes, even fiber! Keto fiber is controversial because it is a carbohydrate, one that the body can't digest on its own, but has many amazing health benefits. So the question becomes, how do you meet your fiber needs in the context of a keto diet?

WHAT IS FIBER?

Fiber, very simply, is a carbohydrate that your body doesn't have the enzymes to break down, so it isn't absorbed into the body as glucose. Soluble fiber passes through and absorbs water to provide bulk and help you to feel full. Insoluble fiber helps your digestive system stay on a regular rhythm. There are also specific prebiotic fibers found in certain foods that actually feed the beneficial bacteria in your colon, balancing the microbiome. Fiber is found in plant foods and eating fiber-rich foods has an array of metabolic benefits, supported by a robust body of research. Diets high in fiber-rich whole foods are associated with longevity, heart health, stable weight, better digestion and overall better metabolic health, including reduced blood sugar and lower cholesterol.

In today's day and age of the industrialized, Standard American Diet, much of the natural fiber has been stripped away leaving high carbohydrates (sugar, flour) without the vitamins, minerals, plant nutrients and fiber the body needs to effectively metabolize the carbs. This food environment characterized by fast, highly processed food is a breeding ground for metabolic syndrome, diabetes, heart disease, weight gain, inflammation and all of the chronic conditions we face in this modern world.

Interestingly, people who move from countries where traditional food systems are still in place, come to the

West and develop these metabolic diseases just as their diet and lifestyles change to meet the new standard diet.

WHY IS FIBER IMPORTANT ON A KETO DIET?

90% of Americans don't eat enough fiber and chances are if you are reading this, you might need to pay a little more attention to fiber, no matter your diet. Specifically, in regards to keto, fiber is key!

For those of you just dipping your toes into keto, a ketogenic diet is one that is high in fat (typically around 75% of daily calories come from fat), moderate protein (15-20%) and low in carbohydrates (5-10%). This macronutrient distribution allows the body to make a metabolic transition from using sugar (glucose) as the primary fuel to using fat in the form of ketones. A ketogenic diet can mimic the metabolic state of our ancestors during times of food scarcity and allow the metabolism to reset.

Although originally used for seizures and neurodegenerative disease, the ketogenic diet holds great promise for weight loss, metabolic syndrome, diabetes, and other chronic, inflammatory conditions.

The traditional keto diet will just focus on the carbohydrate restriction and increasing the fat, instead of paying attention to food quality, nourishment and meeting the body's nutrient needs. Both fiber and a ketogenic diet are beneficial for lowering blood sugar, lowering blood pressure, decreasing weight, improving digestion, supporting the microbiome, taming sugar cravings, reducing inflammation and so much more. By focusing on high fiber, yet low carbohydrate foods along with including good fats and high-quality protein, not only will keto be more satisfying and delicious, but you will also 10X your metabolic benefits.

THE RIGHT WAY TO GO KETO

Focus on fiber.

"If you don't get enough fiber, you don't get all the benefits of nutritional ketosis, consuming fiber while on keto can "speed up your metabolism, balance your hormones, and keep you feeling full." The key is to get your fiber (the FDA recommends 25 grams a day) from non-starchy vegetables, nuts, seeds, and berries instead of traditional high-fiber foods like grains, beans, and legumes.

Eat hydrating foods.

Hydration is even more crucial when you're on a ketogenic diet, explains, because your body is shedding that water that's attached to stored glycogen in your muscles. While drinking H20 is important so is incorporating hydrating foods. Drinking bone broth, adding chia seeds to smoothies and salads, and cooking with unsweetened coconut and coconut oil can also add structured water (which is more dense than regular tap water) to your diet and help keep you hydrated.

Up your electrolyte intake.

The body's transition from burning carbohydrates to fat (and its by-product, ketones) for fuel can sometimes result in the "keto flu," a collection of symptoms that includes dizziness, lack of energy, headaches, and brain fog. That's because at the beginning, your body will burn through stored glucose (glycogen), releasing water, sodium, and other electrolytes. This will cause your insulin levels to drop, and make your kidneys shed even more sodium and water.

Be aware of stress.
It turns out that stress can take you out of nutritional ketosis. When you're in fight or flight mode, your body doesn't produce the same amount of ketones and will start grabbing glucose from the body. On a physical level, coming out of ketosis may make you feel fatigued and foggy with carb cravings. Constant high cortisol leads to muscle loss, and since muscle burns more fuel, you end up with reduced metabolic power.

Don't overdo it on protein.
"People on a keto diet oftentimes eat high protein, but they might actually not be getting enough fat. A keto diet isn't high in protein, but calls for only a moderate amount, or 20 to 25 percent of calories from protein, compared to 65 to 75 percent from fat. "When we over consume protein, that protein will turn into glucose and offset nutritional ketosis.

Why Keto Can Make You Constipated or Give You Diarrhea — and How to Deal
Thing is, most Americans don't get enough of the GI-friendly nutrient anyway. Rule out most sources of carbohydrates, including whole grains, fruits, and legumes, and it's even more likely you'll fall short. Skimping on fiber isn't good for your digestive health, as it feeds the good bacteria in your GI tract, something that benefits you

beyond adequate bowel movements. The digestive tract is where your body's second brain is, and it's home to the majority of your immune system, If you're following keto, it should be one of your biggest priorities to make sure you get adequate fiber to keep your gut healthy and happy, high-fat diets slow digestion and decrease GI motility, so it's especially important to get enough.

What's more, for people with certain health conditions, like diverticulitis, getting ample fiber is necessary to decrease risk of attacks. If you're on certain drugs, like proton pump inhibitors for heartburn, you may also notice changes in your digestion when transitioning to a high-fat diet.

THE 10 BEST SOURCES OF FIBER ON THE KETO DIET

Avocado

All keto followers should consume avocados, as they're a great source of fiber and fat. One avocado contains less than four net carbs, but a whopping 13.5 g of fiber.

Chia Seeds

One ounce (oz) of chia seeds offers 10 g of fiber (and a net carbs total of 2 g). You can make chia seed pudding; lend chia to a small, low-carb smoothie; or sprinkle it onto eggs or a salad.

Pecans

Nuts can be a great option on the keto diet, as they offer a source of fiber and fat. But pecans are one of the lowest-carb nuts, offering just 1 net carb per oz (19 halves). That amount will also supply about 3 g of fiber.

Almonds

That said, almonds are one of the most fiber-rich nuts, clocking in at 3.5 g (and about 2.5 g of net carbs) per oz (23 whole kernels).

Flaxseed

These make a killer crunchy coating for fish or chicken in

lieu of breading. To properly absorb the nutrients in flax, make sure they're ground. One tablespoon of ground flax boasts 2 g of fiber and 0 net carbs. Basically, a freebie eat up.

Collard Greens

Don't swear off all veggies; rather, target high-fiber nonstarchy picks. Greens, like collards, fit the bill. They cook down nicely, so go for greens cooked rather than raw to get in more fiber per cup. One cup of cooked, chopped collards has 3 g of net carbs and nearly 8 g of fiber.

Cauliflower

Cauliflower rice is having a moment and that's great for keto diet followers. A 1-cup serving of this low-carb veggie has only about 3 net carbs and 2 g of fiber. And it's eminently versatile. It can be used to make cauliflower pizza crust, chopped small to stand in for rice, mashed to replace mashed potatoes, and blended into creamy soups.

Raw Coconut

A small piece of coconut meat has about 3 g of net carbs and 4 g of fiber. Plus, it goes double duty to help you get more fats

Pumpkin Seeds

One oz of pumpkin seed kernels yields a little more than 1 g of net carbs, and nearly 2 g of fiber. Plus, they're simple to grab as a handful for a snack, so you can sneak in a bit more fiber into your day.

Green Smoothies

Go ahead and combine a few on this list for a fiber-packed smoothie. Tossing in frozen spinach, zucchini, or cauliflower (like cauliflower rice) adds fiber, vitamins, and minerals for a respectable amount of carbs.

While veggies like zucchini or cauliflower seem like strange smoothie additions, they impart a creamy texture without a strong vegetable taste. Chia seeds also make great smoothie ingredients. Just go easy on the size of the smoothie to not overdo it on the carbs and kick yourself out of ketosis.

ONE LAST THING ABOUT GETTING ENOUGH FIBER ON THE KETO DIET

Fiber is important for everyone, regardless of whether you're on the keto diet. If you're going keto, your best and safest course of action is to enlist a registered dietitian knowledgeable in the diet to design a plan that will meet your nutrient needs. Constipation is considered having fewer than three bowel movements a week, or stools that are hard and dry or difficult to pass, per the NIH. If increasing fiber intake, drinking more water, and being physically active don't help move things along, talk to your doctor.

RECEPIES

ROQUEFORT PEAR SALAD

Ingredients

1 head leaf lettuce, torn into bite-size pieces3 pears - peeled, cored and chopped

5 ounces Roquefort cheese, crumbled

1 avocado - peeled, pitted, and diced

1/2 cup thinly sliced green onions

1/4 cup white sugar

1/2 cup pecans

1/3 cup olive oil

3 tablespoons red wine vinegar

1 1/2 teaspoons white sugar

1 1/2 teaspoons prepared mustard

1 clove garlic, chopped

1/2 teaspoon salt

Fresh ground black pepper to taste

Directions

In a skillet over medium heat, stir 1/4 cup of sugar together with the pecans. Continue stirring gently until sugar has melted and caramelized the pecans.

Carefully transfer nuts onto waxed paper. Allow to cool, and break into pieces.

For the dressing, blend oil, vinegar, 1 1/2 teaspoons sugar, mustard, chopped garlic, salt, and pepper.

In a large serving bowl, layer lettuce, pears, blue cheese, avocado, and green onions. Pour dressing over salad, sprinkle with pecans, and serve.

Nutrition Facts Per Serving:

426 calories; 31.6 g fat; 33.1 g carbohydrates; 8 g protein; 21 mg cholesterol; 654 mg sodium.

MEXICAN BEAN SALAD

Ingredients

1 (15 ounce) can black beans, rinsed and drained

1 (15 ounce) can kidney beans, drained

1 (15 ounce) can cannellini beans, drained and rinsed

1 green bell pepper, chopped

1 red bell pepper, chopped

1 (10 ounce) package frozen corn kernels

1 red onion, chopped

1/2 cup olive oil

1/2 cup red wine vinegar

2 tablespoons fresh lime juice

1 tablespoon lemon juice

2 tablespoons white sugar

1 tablespoon salt

1 clove crushed garlic

1/4 cup chopped fresh cilantro

1/2 tablespoon ground cumin

1/2 tablespoon ground black pepper

1 dash hot pepper sauce

1/2 teaspoon chili powder

Directions

In a large bowl, combine beans, bell peppers, frozen corn, and red onion.

In a small bowl, whisk together olive oil, red wine vinegar, lime juice, lemon juice, sugar, salt, garlic, cilantro, cumin, and black pepper. Season to taste with hot sauce and chili powder.

Pour olive oil dressing over vegetables; mix well. Chill thoroughly, and serve cold.

Nutrition Facts Per Serving:

334 calories; 14.8 g fat; 41.7 g carbohydrates; 11.2 g protein; 0 mg cholesterol; 1159 mg sodium.

KETO CHEESECAKE CUPCAKES

Ingredients

½ cup almond meal

¼ cup butter, melted

2 (8 ounce) packages cream cheese, softened

2 large eggs eggs

¾ cup granular no-calorie sucralose sweetener (such as Splenda®)

1 teaspoon vanilla extract

Directions

Step 1

Preheat oven to 350 degrees F (175 degrees C). Line 12 muffin cups with paper liners.

Step 2

Mix almond meal and butter together in a bowl; spoon into the bottoms of the paper liners and press into a flat crust.

Step 3

Beat cream cheese, eggs, sweetener, and vanilla extract together in a bowl with an electric mixer set to medium until smooth; spoon over the crust layer in the paper liners.

Step 4

Bake in the preheated oven until the cream cheese mixture is nearly set in the middle, 15 to 17 minutes.

Step 5

Let cupcakes cool at room temperature until cool enough to handle. Refrigerate 8 hours to overnight before serving.

Nutrition Facts Per Serving:

208.8 calories; 4.9 g protein; 3.5 g carbohydrates; 82.2 mg cholesterol; 151.1 mg sodium.

APPLE PIE BY GRANDMA OPLE

Ingredients

1 recipe pastry for a 9 inch double crust pie

1/2 cup unsalted butter

3 tablespoons all-purpose flour

1/4 cup water

1/2 cup white sugar

1/2 cup packed brown sugar

8 Granny Smith apples - peeled, cored and sliced

Directions

Preheat oven to 425 degrees F (220 degrees C). Melt the butter in a saucepan. Stir in flour to form a paste. Add water, white sugar and brown sugar, and bring to a boil. Reduce temperature and let simmer.

Place the bottom crust in your pan. Fill with apples, mounded slightly. Cover with a lattice work crust. Gently pour the sugar and butter liquid over the crust. Pour slowly so that it does not run off.

Bake 15 minutes in the preheated oven. Reduce the temperature to 350 degrees F (175 degrees C). Continue baking for 35 to 45 minutes, until apples are soft.

Nutrition Facts per Serving:

512 calories; 26.7 g fat; 67.8 g carbohydrates; 3.6 g protein; 31 mg cholesterol; 241 mg sodium.

SARAH'S APPLESAUCE

Ingredients

4 apples - peeled, cored and chopped

3/4 cup water

1/4 cup white sugar

1/2 teaspoon ground cinnamon

Directions

In a saucepan, combine apples, water, sugar, and cinnamon. Cover, and cook over medium heat for 15 to 20 minutes, or until apples are soft. Allow to cool, then mash with a fork or potato masher.

Nutrition Facts Per Serving:

121 calories; 0.2 g fat; 31.8 g carbohydrates; 0.4 g protein; 0 mg cholesterol; 3 mg sodium.

ANNIE'S FRUIT SALSA AND CINNAMON CHIPS

Ingredients

2 kiwis, peeled and diced

2 Golden Delicious apples - peeled, cored and diced

8 ounces raspberries

1 pound strawberries

2 tablespoons white sugar

1 tablespoon brown sugar

3 tablespoons fruit preserves, any flavor 10 (10 inch) flour

Tortillas butter flavored cooking spray

2 tablespoons cinnamon sugar

Directions

In a large bowl, thoroughly mix kiwis, Golden Delicious apples, raspberries, strawberries, white sugar, brown sugar and fruit preserves. Cover and chill in the refrigerator at least 15 minutes.

Preheat oven to 350 degrees F (175 degrees C).

Coat one side of each flour tortilla with butter flavored cooking spray. Cut into wedges and arrange in a single layer on a large baking sheet. Sprinkle wedges with desired amount of cinnamon sugar. Spray again with cooking spray.

Bake in the preheated oven 8 to 10 minutes. Repeat with any remaining tortilla wedges. Allow to cool approximately 15 minutes. Serve with chilled fruit mixture.

Nutrition Facts Per Serving:

312 calories; 5.9 g fat; 59 g carbohydrates; 6.8 g protein; 0 mg cholesterol; 462 mg sodium.

EASY KETO ALFREDO SAUCE

Ingredient

½ cup unsalted butter

2 cloves garlic, crushed

2 cups heavy whipping cream

½ (4 ounce) package cream cheese, softened

1 ½ cups grated Parmesan cheese

1 pinch salt, or to taste

1 pinch ground nutmeg, or to taste

1 pinch ground white pepper, or to taste

Directions

Step 1

Melt butter in a medium saucepan. Cook garlic until fragrant, about 2 minutes. Add heavy cream and cream cheese. Slowly add Parmesan cheese, stirring constantly until well incorporated and sauce thickens, 5 to 7 minutes. Stir in salt, nutmeg, and white pepper.

Nutrition Facts per Serving:

531.3 calories; 10.3 g protein; 3.8 g carbohydrates; 177.3 mg cholesterol; 391.9 mg sodium.

90-SECOND KETO BREAD IN A MUG

Ingredients

1 tablespoon butter

⅓ cup blanched almond flour

1 egg

½ teaspoon baking powder

1 pinch salt

Directions

STEP 1

Place butter in a microwave-safe mug. Microwave until melted, about 15 seconds. Swirl mug until fully coated.

STEP 2

Combine almond flour, egg, baking powder, and salt in the mug; whisk until smooth.

Step 3

Microwave at maximum power until set, about 90 seconds. Let cool for 2 minutes before slicing.

Nutrition Fact Per Serving:

408 calories; 14.5 g protein; 9.8 g carbohydrates; 194.2 mg cholesterol; 542.2 mg sodium.

ALL-AROUND GOOD SMOOTHIE

Ingredients

1/2 cup nonfat milk

1/2 cup fat-free plain yogurt

1/2 frozen banana, peeled and chopped

2 tablespoons powdered protein supplement

1 1/2 tablespoons flax seed

1 teaspoon honey

1/2 cup frozen strawberries

Directions

In a blender, blend the milk, yogurt, banana, protein supplement, flax seed, honey, and strawberries until smooth.

Nutrition Facts Per Serving:

345 calories; 5.6 g fat; 55.9 g carbohydrates; 26.2 g protein; 5 mg cholesterol; 271 mg sodium.

STRAWBERRY SPINACH SALAD I

Ingredients

2 tablespoons sesame seeds

1 tablespoon poppy seeds

½ cup white sugar

½ cup olive oil

¼ cup distilled white vinegar

¼ teaspoon paprika

¼ teaspoon Worcestershire sauce

1 tablespoon minced onion

10 ounces fresh spinach - rinsed, dried and torn into bite-size pieces

1 quart strawberries - cleaned, hulled and sliced

¼ cup almonds, blanched and slivered

Directions

Step 1

In a medium bowl, whisk together the sesame seeds, poppy seeds, sugar, olive oil, vinegar, paprika, Worcestershire sauce and onion. Cover, and chill for one hour.

Step 2

In a large bowl, combine the spinach, strawberries and almonds. Pour dressing over salad, and toss. Refrigerate 10 to 15 minutes before serving.

Nutrition Facts Per Serving:

490.8 calories; 6 g protein; 42.9 g carbohydrates; 0 mg cholesterol; 62.9 mg sodium.

PEPPERED SHRIMP ALFREDO

Ingredients

12 ounces penne pasta

¼ cup butter

2 tablespoons extra-virgin olive oil

1 onion, diced

2 cloves garlic, minced

1 red bell pepper, diced

½ pound portobello mushrooms, diced

1 pound medium shrimp, peeled and deveined

1 (15 ounce) jar Alfredo sauce

½ cup grated Romano cheese

½ cup cream

1 teaspoon cayenne pepper, or more to taste

1 pinch Salt and pepper to taste

¼ cup chopped parsley

Step 1

Bring a large pot of lightly salted water to a boil. Add pasta and cook for 8 to 10 minutes or until al dente; drain.

Step 2

Meanwhile, melt butter together with the olive oil in a saucepan over medium heat. Stir in onion, and cook until softened and translucent, about 2 minutes. Stir in garlic, red pepper, and mushroom; cook over medium-high heat until soft, about 2 minutes more.

STEP 3

Stir in the shrimp, and cook until firm and pink, then pour in Alfredo sauce, Romano cheese, and cream; bring to a simmer stirring constantly until thickened, about 5 minutes. Season with cayenne, salt, and pepper to taste. Stir drained pasta into the sauce, and serve sprinkled with chopped parsley.

Nutrition Facts Per Serving:

707 calories; 28.4 g protein; 50.6 g carbohydrates; 201.5 mg cholesterol; 1034.5 mg sodium.

DEBDOOZIE'S BLUE RIBBON CHILI

Ingredients

2 pounds ground beef

½ onion, chopped

1 teaspoon ground black pepper

½ teaspoon garlic salt

2 ½ cups tomato sauce

1 (8 ounce) jar salsa

4 tablespoons chili seasoning mix

1 (15 ounce) can light red kidney beans

1 (15 ounce) can dark red kidney beans

Directions

Step 1

In a large saucepan over medium heat, combine the ground beef and the onion and saute for 10 minutes, or until meat is browned and onion is tender. Drain grease, if desired

STEP 2

Add the ground black pepper, garlic salt, tomato sauce, salsa, chili seasoning mix and kidney beans. Mix well, reduce heat to low and simmer for at least an hour.

Nutrition Facts Per Serving:

480.2 calories; 26.7 g protein; 24.9 g carbohydrates; 96.5 mg cholesterol; 1366.2 mg sodium.

CAESAR SALAD SUPREME

Ingredients

6 cloves garlic, peeled, divided

3/4 cup mayonnaise 5 anchovy fillets, minced

6 tablespoons grated Parmesan cheese, divided

1 teaspoon Worcestershire sauce

1 teaspoon Dijon mustard

1 tablespoon lemon juice, or more to taste

Salt to taste

Ground black pepper to taste

1/4 cup olive oil

4 cups day-old bread, cubed

1 head romaine lettuce, torn into bite-size pieces

Directions

Mince 3 cloves of garlic, and combine in a small bowl with mayonnaise, anchovies, 2 tablespoons of the Parmesan cheese, Worcestershire sauce, mustard, and lemon juice. Season to taste with salt and black pepper. Refrigerate until ready to use.

Heat oil in a large skillet over medium heat. Cut the remaining 3 cloves of garlic into quarters, and add to hot oil. Cook and stir until brown, and then remove garlic from pan.

Add bread cubes to the hot oil. Cook, turning frequently, until lightly browned. Remove bread cubes from oil, and season with salt and pepper.

BEET SALAD WITH GOAT CHEESE

Ingredients

4 medium beets - scrubbed, trimmed and cut in half

1/3 cup chopped walnuts

3 tablespoons maple syrup

1 (10 ounce) package mixed baby salad greens

1/2 cup frozen orange juice concentrate

1/4 cup balsamic vinegar

1/2 cup extra-virgin olive oil

2 ounces goat cheese

Directions

Place beets into a saucepan, and fill with enough water to cover. Bring to a boil, then cook for 20 to 30 minutes, until tender. Drain and cool, then cut in to cubes.

While the beets are cooking, place the walnuts in a skillet over medium-low heat. Heat until warm and starting to toast, then stir in the maple syrup. Cook and stir until evenly coated, then remove from the heat and set aside to cool.

In a small bowl, whisk together the orange juice

concentrate, balsamic vinegar and olive oil to make the dressing.

Place a large helping of baby greens onto each of four salad plates, divide candied walnuts equally and sprinkle over the greens. Place equal amounts of beets over the greens, and top with dabs of goat cheese.

Drizzle each plate with some of the dressing.

Nutrition Facts Per Serving:

347 calories; 26.1 g fat; 25 g carbohydrates; 5.3 g protein; 7 mg cholesterol; 107 mg sodium. Full nutrition

AMERICAN POTATO SALAD

Ingredients

5 pounds red potatoes

6 large eggs eggs

2 cups mayonnaise

1 onion, diced

2 medium (4-1/8" long)s green onions, thinly sliced

1 small green bell pepper, seeded and diced

3 stalks celery, thinly sliced

2 teaspoons salt

1 teaspoon ground black pepper

Directions

Step 1

Bring a large pot of water to a boil. Add potatoes, and cook for 15 to 20 minutes, or until tender but still firm. Drain, cool and cut into cubes.

Step 2

Place eggs in a saucepan and cover with cold water. Bring water to a boil and immediately remove from heat. Cover and let eggs stand in hot water for 10 to 12 minutes.

Remove from hot water, cool, peel and chop.

STEP 3

In a large bowl, combine chopped potatoes and eggs. Mix together mayonnaise, chopped onion, green onion, green pepper, and celery. Season with salt and pepper, then mix well. Cover, and refrigerate for several hours or overnight.

Nutrition Facts Per Serving:

328.8 calories; 7.4 g protein; 41.4 g carbohydrates; 103.2 mg cholesterol; 721.4 mg sodium.

BOILERMAKER TAILGATE CHILI

Ingredients

2 pounds ground beef chuck

1 pound bulk Italian sausage

3 (15 ounce) cans chili beans, drained

1 (15 ounce) can chili beans in spicy sauce

2 (28 ounce) cans diced tomatoes with juice

1 (6 ounce) can tomato paste

1 large yellow onion, chopped

3 stalks celery, chopped

1 green bell pepper, seeded and chopped

1 red bell pepper, seeded and chopped

2 green chile peppers, seeded and chopped

1 tablespoon bacon bits

4 cubes beef bouillon

1/2 cup beer

1/4 cup chili powder

1 tablespoon Worcestershire sauce

1 tablespoon minced garlic

1 tablespoon dried oregano

2 teaspoons ground cumin

2 teaspoons hot pepper sauce (e.g. Tabasco™)

1 teaspoon dried basil

1 teaspoon salt

1 teaspoon ground black pepper

1 teaspoon cayenne pepper

1 teaspoon paprika

1 teaspoon white sugar

1 (10.5 ounce) bag corn chips such as Fritos®

1 (8 ounce) package shredded Cheddar cheese

Directions

Heat a large stock pot over medium-high heat. Crumble the ground chuck and sausage into the hot pan, and cook until evenly browned. Drain off excess grease.

Pour in the chili beans, spicy chili beans, diced tomatoes and tomato paste. Add the onion, celery, green and red bell peppers, chile peppers, bacon bits, bouillon, and beer. Season with chili powder, Worcestershire sauce, garlic, oregano, cumin, hot pepper sauce, basil, salt, pepper, cayenne, paprika, and sugar. Stir to blend, then cover and simmer over low heat for at least 2 hours, stirring occasionally.

After 2 hours, taste, and adjust salt, pepper, and chili powder if necessary. The longer the chili simmers, the better it will taste. Remove from heat and serve, or refrigerate, and serve the next day.

To serve, ladle into bowls, and top with corn chips and shredded Cheddar cheese.

Nutrition Facts Per Serving:

600 calories; 30.1 g fat; 55.3 g carbohydrates; 30.8 g protein; 70 mg cholesterol; 2092 mg sodium.

FLATLANDER CHILI

Ingredients

2 pounds lean ground beef

1 (46 fluid ounce) can tomato juice

1 (29 ounce) can tomato sauce

1 1/2 cups chopped onion

1/2 cup chopped celery

1/4 cup chopped green bell Pepper

1/4 cup chili powder

2 teaspoons ground cumin

1 1/2 teaspoons garlic powder

1 teaspoon salt

1/2 teaspoon ground black pepper

1/2 teaspoon dried oregano

1/2 teaspoon white sugar

1/8 teaspoon ground cayenne pepper

2 cups canned red beans, drained and rinsed

Directions

Place ground beef in a large, deep skillet. Cook over medium-high heat until evenly brown. Drain, crumble, and set aside.

Add all ingredients to a large kettle. Bring to boil. Reduce heat and simmer for 1 to 1 1/2 hours, stirring occasionally.

Nutrition Facts Per Serving:

347 calories; 19.9 g fat; 22.6 g carbohydrates; 21.4 g protein; 68 mg cholesterol; 1246 mg sodium.

PUMPKIN TURKEY CHILI

Ingredients

1 tablespoon vegetable oil

1 cup chopped onion

1/2 cup chopped green bell pepper

1/2 cup chopped yellow bell pepper

1 clove garlic, minced

1 pound ground turkey

1 (14.5 ounce) can diced tomatoes

2 cups pumpkin puree

1 1/2 tablespoons chili powder

1/2 teaspoon ground black pepper

1 dash salt

1/2 cup shredded Cheddar cheese

1/2 cup sour cream

Directions

Heat the oil in a large skillet over medium heat, and saute the onion, green bell pepper, yellow bell pepper, and garlic until tender. Stir in the turkey, and cook until evenly brown. Drain, and mix in tomatoes and pumpkin. Season with chili powder, pepper, and salt. Reduce heat to low, cover, and simmer 20 minutes. Serve topped with Cheddar cheese and sour cream.

Nutrition Facts Per Serving:

285 calories; 16.6 g fat; 14.9 g carbohydrates; 21.2 g protein; 76 mg cholesterol; 321 mg sodium.

BUTTERNUT SQUASH AND TURKEY CHILI

Ingredients

2 tablespoons olive oil

1 onion, chopped

2 cloves garlic, minced

1 pound ground turkey breast

1 pound butternut squash - peeled, seeded and cut into 1-inch dice

½ cup chicken broth

1 (4.5 ounce) can chopped green chilies

2 (14.5 ounce) cans petite diced tomatoes

1 (15 ounce) can kidney beans with liquid

1 (15.5 ounce) can white hominy, drained

1 (8 ounce) can tomato sauce

1 tablespoon chili powder

1 tablespoon ground cumin

1 teaspoon garlic salt

Directions

STEP 1

Heat the olive oil in a large pot over medium heat. Stir in the onion and garlic; cook and stir for 3 minutes, then add the turkey, and stir until crumbly and no longer pink.

Step 2

Add the butternut squash, chicken broth, green chilies, tomatoes, kidney beans, hominy, and tomato sauce; season with chili powder, cumin, and garlic salt. Bring to a simmer, then reduce heat to medium-low, cover, and simmer until the squash is tender, about 20 minutes.

Nutrition Facts Per Serving:

165 calories; 13.4 g protein; 20.5 g carbohydrates; 23.7 mg cholesterol; 709.2 mg sodium.

KETO CHICKEN PARMESAN

Ingredients

1 (8 ounce) skinless, boneless chicken breast

1 egg

1 tablespoon heavy whipping cream

1 ½ ounces pork rinds, crushed

1 ounce grated Parmesan cheese

½ teaspoon salt

½ teaspoon garlic powder

½ teaspoon red pepper flakes

½ teaspoon ground black pepper

½ teaspoon Italian seasoning

½ cup jarred tomato sauce

¼ cup shredded mozzarella cheese

1 tablespoon ghee (clarified butter)

Directions

Step 1

Set oven rack about 6 inches from the heat source and preheat the oven's broiler.

Step 2

Slice chicken breast through the middle horizontally from one side to within 1/2 inch of the other side. Open the two sides and spread them out like an open book.

Step 3

Beat egg and cream together in a bowl.

Step 4

Combine crushed pork rinds, Parmesan cheese, salt, garlic powder, red pepper flakes, ground black pepper, and Italian seasoning in bowl; transfer breading to a plate.

Step 5

Dip chicken into egg mixture; coat completely. Press chicken into breading; thickly coat both sides.

Step 6

Heat a skillet over medium-high heat; add ghee. Place chicken in the pan; cook until no longer pink in the center and the juices run clear, about 3 minutes per side. An instant-read thermometer inserted into the center should read at least 165 degrees F (74 degrees C). Be careful to keep breading in place.

Step 7

Transfer chicken to a baking sheet. Cover with tomato sauce; top with mozzarella cheese.

Step 8

Broil until cheese is bubbling and barely browned, about 2 minutes.

Nutrition Facts Per Serving:

441.5 calories; 46.5 g protein; 5.8 g carbohydrates; 216.8 mg cholesterol; 1604.7 mg sodium.

GUACAMOLE

Ingredients

3 avocados - peeled, pitted, and mashed

1 lime, juiced

1 teaspoon salt

1/2 cup diced onion

3 tablespoons chopped fresh cilantro

2 roma (plum) tomatoes, diced

1 teaspoon minced garlic

1 pinch ground cayenne pepper (optional)

Directions

In a medium bowl, mash together the avocados, lime juice, and salt. Mix in onion, cilantro, tomatoes, and garlic. Stir in cayenne pepper. Refrigerate 1 hour for best flavor, or serve immediately.

Nutrition Facts Per Serving:

262 calories; 22.2 g fat; 18 g carbohydrates; 3.7 g protein; 0 mg cholesterol; 596 mg sodium.

EASY GUACAMOLE

Ingredients

2 avocado, NS as to Florida or Californias avocados

1 small onion, finely chopped

1 clove garlic, minced

1 ripe tomato, chopped

1 lime, juiced

Directions

Step 1

Peel and mash avocados in a medium serving bowl. Stir in onion, garlic, tomato, lime juice, salt and pepper. Season with remaining lime juice and salt and pepper to taste. Chill for half an hour to blend flavors.

Nutrition Facts Per Serving:

44.9 calories; 0.7 g protein; 3.4 g carbohydrates; 0 mg cholesterol; 2.4 mg sodium. Full Nutrition

Seven Layer Dip II
Ingredients

2 avocados - peeled, pitted and diced

1 1/2 tablespoons fresh lime juice

1/4 cup chopped fresh cilantro

1/4 cup salsagarlic salt to taste ground black pepper to taste

1 (8 ounce) container sour cream

1 (1 ounce) package taco seasoning mix

4 roma (plum) tomatoes, diced

1 bunch green onions, finely chopped

1 (16 ounce) can refried beans

2 cups shredded Mexican-style cheese blend

1 (2.25 ounce) can black olives - drained and finely chopped

Directions
In a medium bowl, mash the avocados. Mix in lime juice, cilantro, salsa, garlic salt and pepper.

In a small bowl, blend the sour cream and taco seasoning.

In a 9x13 inch dish or on a large serving platter, spread the refried beans. Top with sour cream mixture. Spread on guacamole. Top with tomatoes, green onions, Mexican-style cheese blend and black olives.

Nutrition Facts Per Serving:

42 calories; 2.9 g fat; 2.8 g carbohydrates; 1.5 g protein; 5 mg cholesterol; 92 mg sodium.

Tangy Cucumber and Avocado Salad
Ingredients
2 medium cucumbers, cubed

2 avocados, cubed

4 tablespoons chopped fresh cilantro

1 clove garlic, minced

2 tablespoons minced green onions (optional)

1/4 teaspoon saltblack pepper to taste

1/4 large lemon1 lime

Directions

In a large bowl, combine cucumbers, avocados, and cilantro. Stir in garlic, onions, salt, and pepper. Squeeze lemon and lime over the top, and toss. Cover, and refrigerate at least 30 minutes.

Nutrition Facts Per Serving:

186 calories; 14.9 g fat; 15.5 g carbohydrates; 3.1 g protein; 0 mg cholesterol; 157 mg sodium.

AVOCADO MANGO SALSA

Ingredients

1 avocado - peeled, pitted and diced

1 lime, juiced

1 mango - peeled, seeded and diced

1 small red onion, chopped

1 habanero pepper, seeded and chopped

1 tablespoon chopped fresh cilantrosalt to taste

Directions

Place the avocado in a serving bowl, and mix with the lime juice. Mix in the mango, onion, habanero pepper, cilantro and salt.

Nutrition Facts Per Serving:

63 calories; 3.8 g fat; 8.3 g carbohydrates; 0.8 g protein; 0 mg cholesterol; 3 mg sodium.

ITALIAN SAUSAGE SOUP

Ingredients

1 pound Italian sausage

1 clove garlic, minced

2 (14 ounce) cans beef broth

1 (14.5 ounce) can Italian-style stewed tomatoes

1 cup sliced carrots1 (14.5 ounce) can great Northern beans, undrained

2 small zucchini, cubed

2 cups spinach - packed, rinsed and torn

1/4 teaspoon ground black pepper

1/4 teaspoon salt

Directions

In a stockpot or Dutch oven, brown sausage with garlic. Stir in broth, tomatoes and carrots, and season with salt and pepper. Reduce heat, cover, and simmer 15 minutes.

Stir in beans with liquid and zucchini. Cover, and simmer another 15 minutes, or until zucchini is tender.

Remove from heat, and add spinach. Replace lid allowing the heat from the soup to cook the spinach leaves. Soup is ready to serve after 5 minutes.

Nutrition Facts Per Serving:

385 calories; 24.4 g fat; 22.5 g carbohydrates; 18.8 g
protein; 58 mg cholesterol; 1259 mg sodium

ITALIAN SAUSAGE SOUP WITH TORTELLINI

Ingredients

1 pound sweet Italian sausage, casings removed

1 cup chopped onion

2 cloves garlic, minced

5 cups beef broth

1/2 cup water

1/2 cup red wine

4 large tomatoes - peeled, seeded and chopped

1 cup thinly sliced carrots

1/2 tablespoon packed fresh basil leaves

1/2 teaspoon dried oregano

1 (8 ounce) can tomato sauce

1 1/2 cups sliced zucchini 8 ounces fresh tortellini pasta

3 tablespoons chopped fresh parsley

Directions

In a 5 quart Dutch oven, brown sausage. Remove sausage and drain, reserving 1 tablespoon of the drippings.

Saute onions and garlic in drippings. Stir in beef broth, water, wine, tomatoes, carrots, basil, oregano, tomato sauce, and sausage. Bring to a boil. Reduce heat; simmer uncovered for 30 minutes.

Skim fat from the soup. Stir in zucchini and parsley. Simmer covered for 30 minutes. Add tortellini during the last 10 minutes. Sprinkle with Parmesan cheese on top of each serving.

Nutrition Facts Per Serving:

324 calories; 20.2 g fat; 19.1 g carbohydrates; 14.6 g protein; 50 mg cholesterol; 1145 mg sodium.

ITALIAN SAUSAGE, PEPPERS, AND ONIONS

Ingredients

6 (4 ounce) links sweet Italian sausage

2 tablespoons butter

1 yellow onion, sliced

1/2 red onion, sliced

4 cloves garlic, minced

1 large red bell pepper, sliced

1 green bell pepper, sliced

1 teaspoon dried basil

1 teaspoon dried oregano

1/4 cup white wine

Directions

Place the sausage in a large skillet over medium heat, and brown on all sides. Remove from skillet, and slice.

Melt butter in the skillet. Stir in the yellow onion, red onion, and garlic, and cook 2 to 3 minutes. Mix in red bell pepper and green bell pepper. Season with basil, and oregano. Stir in white wine. Continue to cook and stir until peppers and onions are tender.

Return sausage slices to skillet with the vegetables. Reduce heat to low, cover, and simmer 15 minutes, or until sausage is heated through.

Nutrition Facts Per Serving:

461 calories; 39.4 g fat; 7 g carbohydrates; 17.1 g protein; 96 mg cholesterol; 857 mg sodium.

SAUSAGE BARLEY SOUP

Ingredients

1 pound Italian sausage

1/2 cup diced onion

1 tablespoon minced garlic

1/2 teaspoon Italian seasoning

1 (48 fluid ounce) can chicken broth

1 large carrot, sliced

1 (10 ounce) package frozen chopped spinach

1/4 cup uncooked pearl barley

Directions

In a skillet over medium heat, cook the sausage, onion, and garlic until the sausage is evenly brown. Season with Italian seasoning. Remove from heat, and drain.

In a slow cooker, mix the sausage mixture, chicken broth, carrot, spinach, and barley.

Cover, and cook 4 hours on High or 6 to 8 hours on Low.

Nutrition Facts Per Serving:

382 calories; 22.9 g fat; 23.2 g carbohydrates; 20.7 g

protein; 54 mg cholesterol; 2722 mg sodium.

HEARTY ITALIAN MEATBALL SOUP

Ingredients

3 cups water

2 (14 ounce) cans diced tomatoes with onion and garlic, undrained

2 (14 ounce) cans beef broth

1 teaspoon Italian seasoning

1 (16 ounce) package frozen cooked Italian-style meatballs

2 cups frozen Italian-blend vegetables

1 cup small star-shaped dried pasta

1/4 cup grated Parmesan cheese

Directions

Stir water, tomatoes, beef broth, and Italian seasoning together in a large pot; bring to a boil. Add meatballs, Italian-blend vegetables, and pasta to the pot.

Return broth to a boil, reduce heat to medium-low, and cook until the meatballs are heated through and the pasta is tender, about 10 minutes. Ladle soup into bowls and garnish with Parmesan cheese.

Nutrition Facts Per Serving:

272 calories; 8.9 g fat; 30.8 g carbohydrates; 16.7 g protein; 49 mg cholesterol; 498 mg sodium. Full nutrition

MEGAN'S GRANOLA

Ingredients

8 cups rolled oats

1 1/2 cups wheat germ

1 1/2 cups oat bran

1 cup sunflower seeds

1 cup finely chopped almonds

1 cup finely chopped pecans

1 cup finely chopped walnuts

1 1/2 teaspoons salt

1/2 cup brown sugar

1/4 cup maple syrup

3/4 cup honey

1 cup vegetable oil

1 tablespoon ground cinnamon

1 tablespoon vanilla extract

2 cups raisins or sweetened dried cranberries

Directions

Preheat the oven to 325 degrees F (165 degrees C). Line two large baking sheets with parchment or aluminum foil.

Combine the oats, wheat germ, oat bran, sunflower seeds, almonds, pecans, and walnuts in a large bowl. Stir together the salt, brown sugar, maple syrup, honey, oil, cinnamon, and vanilla in a saucepan. Bring to a boil over medium heat, then pour over the dry ingredients, and stir to coat. Spread the mixture out evenly on the baking sheets.

Bake in the preheated oven until crispy and toasted, about 20 minutes. Stir once halfway through. Cool, then stir in the raisins or cranberries before storing in an airtight container.

Nutrition Facts Per Serving:

369 calories; 20 g fat; 45 g carbohydrates; 8.3 g protein; 0 mg cholesterol; 122 mg sodium.

PLAYGROUP GRANOLA BARS

Ingredients

2 cups rolled oats

3/4 cup packed brown sugar

1/2 cup wheat germ

3/4 teaspoon ground cinnamon

1 cup all-purpose flour

3/4 cup raisins (optional

3/4 teaspoon salt

1/2 cup honey

1 egg, beaten

1/2 cup vegetable oil

2 teaspoons vanilla extract

Directions

Preheat the oven to 350 degrees F (175 degrees C). Generously grease a 9x13 inch baking pan.

In a large bowl, mix together the oats, brown sugar, wheat germ, cinnamon, flour, raisins and salt. Make a well in the center, and pour in the honey, egg, oil and vanilla. Mix well using your hands. Pat the mixture evenly into the prepared pan.

Bake for 30 to 35 minutes in the preheated oven, until the bars begin to turn golden at the edges. Cool for 5 minutes, then cut into bars while still warm. Do not allow the bars to cool completely before cutting, or they will be too hard to cut.

Nutrition Facts Per Serving:

161 calories; 5.5 g fat; 26.6 g carbohydrates; 2.4 g protein; 8 mg cholesterol; 79 mg sodium.

OOEY-GOOEY CINNAMON BUNS

Ingredients

1 teaspoon white sugar

1 (.25 ounce) package active dry yeast

1/2 cup warm water (110 degrees F/45 degrees C)

1/2 cup milk

1/4 cup white sugar

1/4 cup butter

1 teaspoon salt

2 eggs, beaten

4 cups all-purpose flour

3/4 cup butter

3/4 cup brown sugar1

cup chopped pecans, divided

3/4 cup brown sugar

1 tablespoon ground cinnamon

1/4 cup melted butter

Directions

In a small bowl, dissolve 1 teaspoon sugar and yeast in warm water. Let stand until creamy, about 10 minutes. Warm the milk in a small saucepan until it bubbles, then remove from heat. Mix in 1/4 cup sugar, 1/4 cup butter and salt; stir until melted. Let cool until lukewarm.

In a large bowl, combine the yeast mixture, milk mixture, eggs and 1 1/2 cup flour; stir well to combine. Stir in the remaining flour, 1/2 cup at a time, beating well after each addition. When the dough has pulled together, turn it out onto a lightly floured surface and knead until smooth and elastic, about 8 minutes.

Lightly oil a large bowl, place the dough in the bowl and turn to coat with oil. Cover with a damp cloth and let rise in a warm place until doubled in volume, about 1 hour.

While dough is rising, melt 3/4 cup butter in a small saucepan over medium heat. Stir in 3/4 cup brown sugar, whisking until smooth. Pour into greased 9x13 inch baking pan. Sprinkle bottom of pan with 1/2 cup pecans; set aside. Melt remaining butter; set aside. Combine remaining 3/4 cup brown sugar, 1/2 cup pecans, and cinnamon; set aside.

Turn dough out onto a lightly floured surface, roll into an 18x14 inch rectangle. Brush with 2 tablespoons melted butter, leaving 1/2 inch border uncovered; sprinkle with brown sugar cinnamon mixture. Starting at long side, tightly roll up, pinching seam to seal. Brush with remaining 2 tablespoons butter. With serrated knife, cut into 15 pieces; place cut side down, in prepared pan. Cover and let rise for 1 hour or until doubled in volume. Meanwhile, preheat oven to 375 degrees F (190 degrees C).

Bake in preheated oven for 25 to 30 minutes, until golden

brown. Let cool in pan for 3 minutes, then invert onto serving platter. Scrape remaining filling from the pan onto the rolls.

Nutrition Facts Per Serving: 392 calories; 21.7 g fat; 45.3 g carbohydrates; 5.6 g protein; 66 mg cholesterol; 282 mg sodium.

OATMEAL PEANUT BUTTER COOKIES III

Ingredients

3/4 cup all-purpose flour

1/2 teaspoon baking soda

1/4 teaspoon baking powder

1/2 teaspoon salt

1/2 cup butter, softened

1/2 cup peanut butter

1/2 cup white sugar

1/2 cup packed light brown sugar1

 egg1 teaspoon vanilla extract

1 cup quick cooking oats

3 tablespoons butter, softened

1 cup confectioners' sugar

1/2 cup smooth peanut butter

2 1/2 tablespoons heavy whipping cream

Directions

In a large bowl, cream together 1/2 cup butter or

margarine, 1/2 cup peanut butter, white sugar, brown sugar, and vanilla. Add egg and beat well.

In another bowl, combine the flour, baking soda, baking powder, and salt. Add these dry ingredients to the creamed mixture. Stir. Add oatmeal and stir.

Drop by teaspoons onto greased baking sheet, and press each mound down with a fork to form 1/4 inch thick cookies. Bake at 350 degrees F (175 degrees C) for 10 minutes, or until cookies are a light brown.

To Make Filling: Cream 3 tablespoons butter or margarine with the confectioners' sugar, 1/2 cup smooth peanut butter, and the cream. Spread filling onto half of the cooled cookies, then top with the other half to form sandwiches.

Nutrition Facts Per Serving:

397 calories; 23.5 g fat; 42.2 g carbohydrates; 7.8 g protein; 48 mg cholesterol; 343 mg sodium.

APPLE RAISIN FRENCH TOAST STRATA

Ingredients

1 (1 pound) loaf cinnamon raisin bread, cubed

1 (8 ounce) package cream cheese, diced

1 cup diced peeled apples

8 eggs

2 1/2 cups half-and-half cream

6 tablespoons butter, melted

1/4 cup maple syrup

Directions

Coat a 9x13 inch baking dish with cooking spray. Arrange 1/2 of the cubed raisin bread in the bottom of the dish. Sprinkle the cream cheese evenly over the bread, and top with the apples. If you like extra raisins, add them now. Top with remaining bread.

In a large bowl, beat the eggs with the cream, butter, and maple syrup. Pour over the bread mixture. Cover with plastic wrap, and press down so that all bread pieces are soaked. Refrigerate at least 2 hours.

Preheat oven to 325 degrees F (165 degrees C).

Bake 45 minutes in the preheated oven. Let stand for 10 minutes before serving.

Nutrition Facts Per Serving:

354 calories; 23.1 g fat; 28.3 g carbohydrates; 10.1 g protein; 178 mg cholesterol; 310 mg sodium.

JAMIE'S CRANBERRY SPINACH SALAD

Ingredients

1 tablespoon butter

¾ cup almonds, blanched and slivered

1 pound spinach, rinsed and torn into bite-size pieces

1 cup dried cranberries

2 tablespoons toasted sesame seeds

1 tablespoon poppy seeds

½ cup white sugar

2 teaspoons minced onion

¼ teaspoon paprika

¼ cup white wine vinegar

¼ cup cider vinegar

½ cup vegetable oil

Directions

STEP 1

In a medium saucepan, melt butter over medium heat. Cook and stir almonds in butter until lightly toasted. Remove from heat, and let cool.

STEP 2

In a medium bowl, whisk together the sesame seeds, poppy seeds, sugar, onion, paprika, white wine vinegar, cider vinegar, and vegetable oil. Toss with spinach just before serving.

STEP 3

In a large bowl, combine the spinach with the toasted almonds and cranberries.

Nutrition Facts Per Serving:

338.2 calories; 4.9 g protein; 30.4 g carbohydrates; 3.8 mg cholesterol; 58.1 mg sodium.

MISSY'S CANDIED WALNUT GORGONZOLA SALAD

Ingredients

½ cup walnut halves

¼ cup sugar

3 cups mixed greens

½ cup dried cranberries

½ cup crumbled Gorgonzola cheese

1 tablespoon raspberry vinaigrette

1 tablespoon white vinegar

1 tablespoon olive oil

Directions

Step 1

Place walnuts and sugar in a skillet over medium heat, stirring constantly until the sugar dissolves into a light brown liquid and coats the walnuts. Remove walnuts from skillet, and spread them out on a sheet of aluminum foil to cool.

ARNOLD KUNTZ PH.D

cool.

STEP 2

Place in a large salad bowl the mixed greens, cranberries, cheese, vinaigrette, vinegar, and olive oil. Toss gently; add candied walnuts, and toss again.

Nutrition Facts Per Serving:

307.7 calories; 7.4 g protein; 29.4 g carbohydrates; 22.5 mg cholesterol; 273.4 mg sodium.

SPINACH AND STRAWBERRY SALAD

Ingredients

2 bunches spinach, rinsed and torn into bite-size pieces

4 cups sliced strawberries

½ cup vegetable oil

¼ cup white wine vinegar

½ cup white sugar

¼ teaspoon paprika

2 tablespoons sesame seeds

1 tablespoon poppy seeds

Directions

STEP 1

In a large bowl, toss together the spinach and strawberries.

Step 2

In a medium bowl, whisk together the oil, vinegar, sugar, paprika, sesame seeds, and poppy seeds. Pour over the spinach and strawberries, and toss to coat.

Nutrition Facts Per Serving:

234.8 calories; 3.6 g protein; 22.8 g carbohydrates; 0 mg cholesterol; 69.3 mg sodium.

STRAWBERRY SPINACH SALAD I

Ingredients

2 tablespoons sesame seeds

1 tablespoon poppy seeds

½ cup white sugar

½ cup olive oil

¼ cup distilled white vinegar

¼ teaspoon paprika

¼ teaspoon Worcestershire sauce

1 tablespoon minced onion

10 ounces fresh spinach - rinsed, dried and torn into bite-size pieces

1 quart strawberries - cleaned, hulled and sliced

¼ cup almonds, blanched and slivered

Directions

STEP 1

In a medium bowl, whisk together the sesame seeds, poppy seeds, sugar, olive oil, vinegar, paprika, Worcestershire sauce and onion. Cover, and chill for one hour.

STEP 2

In a large bowl, combine the spinach, strawberries and almonds. Pour dressing over salad, and toss. Refrigerate 10 to 15 minutes before serving.

Nutrition Facts Per Serving:

490.8 calories; 6 g protein; 42.9 g carbohydrates; 0 mg cholesterol; 62.9 mg sodium.

STRAWBERRY, KIWI, AND SPINACH SALAD

Ingredients

2 tablespoons raspberry vinegar

2 ½ tablespoons raspberry jam

⅓ cup vegetable oil

8 cups spinach, rinsed and torn into bite-size pieces

½ cup chopped walnuts

8 medium (1-1/4" dia)s strawberries, quartered

2 eaches kiwis, peeled and sliced

Step 1

Mix together raspberry vinegar, raspberry jam, and vegetable oil in a small container.

Step 2

Combine spinach, nuts, strawberries, and kiwi in a salad bowl. Toss with raspberry dressing.

Nutrition Facts Per Serving:

168.8 calories; 2.3 g protein; 10.3 g carbohydrates; 0 mg cholesterol; 25.4 mg sodium.

CONCLUSION

One thing that's often missing from the keto diet, a little bit of roughage. The popular diet, which often requires eating up to 80 percent of your calories from fat and only 20 to 50 grams (g) of carbohydrates per day, is often criticized for being distinctly lacking in fiber. And, that's certainly the case for some followers. "A poorly planned keto diet is at risk of being deficient in fiber, dietitians frequently see patients who complain of constipation when they go keto.

www.ingramcontent.com/pod-product-compliance
Lightning Source LLC
Chambersburg PA
CBHW071542150726
48000CB00002B/894